Intermittent Fasting For Weight Loss: A Beginners 7 Step Guide To The 16:8 Diet

Robert Paxton

FREE BONUS

Wait! Claim Your FREE Bonus!

One of the biggest obstacles to success is motivation and support. As promised, I'm giving you **FREE LIFE TIME ACCESS** to my private Facebook group. Here you'll be able to ask me questions directly plus become connected with others on the same journey as you!

Simply visit : **http://bit.ly/fasting_motivation**

Introduction

Hello fellow faster…..

Once upon I time I was in your very shoes….

I was excited to start fasting to <u>FINALLY</u> reach my weight loss goals but a few questions were holding me back.

Is there anything I have to do or protocols I should follow before I actually start IF?

Does it matter what time of day my eating window starts?

Should I be reducing, counting, increasing or tracking my caloric intake?

What is the best exercise to do while fasting for weight loss?

Now there were all kinds of answers to these questions online but a lot of the information was contradictory……..

I ended up having to work it out myself through trial and error….

This meant it took much **LONGER** for me to lose weight than it should have……

I Don't Want This For You!

That's why I created the Short Cut to Start Fasting guide so people like yourself can start **TODAY!**

Now you'll be able to actually <u>START</u> your IF journey with the confidence you're going about it the right way.

Good luck!

© **Copyright 2018 - All rights reserved.**

This document is geared towards providing exact and reliable information in regards to the topic and issue covered. The publication is sold with the idea that the publisher is not required to render accounting, officially permitted, or otherwise, qualified services. If advice is necessary, legal or professional, a practiced individual in the profession should be ordered.

- From a Declaration of Principles which was accepted and approved equally by a Committee of the American Bar Association and a Committee of Publishers and Associations.

In no way is it legal to reproduce, duplicate, or transmit any part of this document in either electronic means or in printed format. Recording of this publication is strictly prohibited and any storage of this document is not allowed unless with written permission from the publisher. All rights reserved.

The information provided herein is stated to be truthful and consistent, in that any liability, in terms of inattention or otherwise, by any usage or abuse of any policies, processes, or directions contained within is the solitary and utter responsibility of the recipient reader. Under no circumstances will any legal responsibility or blame be held against the publisher for any reparation, damages, or monetary loss due to the information herein, either directly or indirectly.

Respective authors own all copyrights not held by the publisher.

The information herein is offered for informational purposes solely, and is universal as so. The presentation of the information is without contract or any type of guarantee assurance.

The trademarks that are used are without any consent, and the publication of the trademark is without permission or backing by the trademark owner. All trademarks and brands within this book are for clarifying purposes only and are the owned by the owners themselves, not affiliated with this document.

Contents

FREEBONUS 2

Chapter 1: What Is Intermittent Fasting? 6

Chapter 2: Selecting An Ideal Eating Window 13

Chapter 3: Protein 20

Chapter 4: Carbohydrates 26

Chapter 5: Healthy Fats 33

Chapter 6: Sugar 39

Chapter 7: How To Break A Fast 44

End Note 47

References 49

Chapter 1: What Is Intermittent Fasting?

Intermittent Fasting (IF) can be described as an eating pattern where a person chooses to abstain from food, and in some cases water for a given period of time. The 16:8 method consists of an eight hour window where a person would consume all their meals and a 16 hour window where they'd consume nothing; perhaps with the exception of 0 calorie drinks such as black coffee.

IF is a choice and for the context of this book a tool for weight loss and better health. Fasting in order to commit to prayer or because of the shear lack of resources are not considered IF or apart of the 16:8 method.

The ability to achieve sustainable weight loss depends on many factors, One often ignored is hormonal balance. The term calories in vs calories out is well known, but interestingly many who try low calorie diets get little to no results. Why? Calories are only half the equation. We are now working harder, sleeping less and eating undesirably more often than we should. Add stress and the processed food industry to complete a cocktail for unfavourable hormonal imbalances; especially when trying to lose weight!

IF methods such as 16:8 have been proven to help reverse these imbalances and help promote positive hormonal adaptations.

Keep reading for a quick overview of how this process works

Energy Storage
The body has the ability to store two sources of energy; glucose and fat. Each process is determined by certain hormones who's secretion is dictated by blood sugar levels.

Glucose (sugar) is the bodies preferred fuel and is utilized faster than fat. Our bodies store glucose as glycogen in the liver and muscles. Once glycogen stores are full however, any excess will be stored as fat.

Fat stores have almost unlimited storage space. The body is primed to save as much as it can in case of famine and scarcity. A necessary skill in ancient times, annoying when trying to lose weight in the modern world. In some cases you will first need to deplete glycogen stores in order to burn fat.

Blood sugar levels determine which hormones are secreted. Hormones responsible for storage are released when blood sugar rises, while their counterparts responsible for breaking down stored energy are released when blood sugar levels drop. For this reason you will never truly be in a state of storage and burning at the same time - regardless of how healthy you eat. This is why the timing of certain food groups can impact what results we get.

Hormones

Our hormones control everything from how we feel to how we burn fat. Following is a short overview of the hormones that control the before mentioned outcomes.

Insulin

Trigger: Secreted when blood sugar or protein levels rise

Function: Lower blood sugar and/or protein levels by prompting cells to absorb glucose and/or amino acids for use. In times of glucose excess, insulin also promotes storage of glycogen and fat.

Human Growth Hormone (HGH)

Trigger: HGH secretion can be triggered by many events including quality sleep and exercise. For the context of fasting, all you need to know is it's secretion is triggered by low blood sugar levels.

Function: Our bodies utilize HGH for a variety of different functions including bone growth in children. In terms of weight loss however, HGH stimulates fat cells to breakdown stored fat when blood sugar levels are low.

Glucagon

Trigger: Like HGH, glucagon is secreted in reaction to low blood sugar levels.

Function: Glucagon stimulates the liver to convert stored glycogen into glucose for the blood stream. It also plays a role in the breakdown of fat in adipose cells.

Why Does Counting Calories Not Work?

"Eat less, move more". It sounds logical right? If I eat less than I burn each day how could I not lose weight? If you're reading this book chances are you've tried this concept and received little to no results...

In fact any results you did get were probably short lived. Keep reading to see how unfavourable eating patterns can cause people to plateau; even in caloric deficit.

Metabolic Adaptation

BMR (basal metabolic rate) or RMR (resting metabolic rate) make up roughly 70% of your entire metabolism. They refer to how many calories your body uses to live without movement. When caloric intake is lowered, the bodies BMR/RMR slowly drops to accommodate the lower number of calories. Basically, your metabolism slows down. This is an important reaction through times of famine. The body doesn't want to use stored energy and naturally uses incoming energy sparingly. This is not beneficial when the aim is sustainable weight loss. When you start dieting in this manner, you'll generally see results at the start before your body's metabolism adjusts for the lack of food. Once it adjusts, your results become stagnant and often times people give up. Once they go back to eating as they did previously all the weight piles back on. Frustrating!

Metabolic syndrome

Metabolic adaptation also occurs if you suddenly start eating normally again. Just like when you cut calories however, your body will take time to adapt. Your lower metabolism will most probably realign right around the time you end up back where you started, Frustrating!

Some studies show constant yo-yo dieting could lead to a lower metabolism permanently or at least for a very long time. Some suggest 10 – 15 years. In fact precision nutrition released a review of a 2014 study done on the hit TV series "The Biggest Loser". The study showed 98% of the contestants had regained most of their starting weight 6 years after the show. The worst thing was their RMR was now lower than when they started. Data showed the contestants RMR naturally dropped as they lost weight but didn't rise and stabilize with weight regain. Now, just to maintain their old weight they'd have to eat less and/or exercise more. A hard feat considering they were exercising for 90 minutes six days a week while consuming around 1500 calories while on the show. Metabolic syndrome could be one reason many struggle to lose weight even under calorie restriction and intense exercise regimes.

Insulin Resistance
As mentioned earlier Insulin is a hormone triggered when blood Glucose (sugar) levels rise. Once released, it will actively work to return these levels too normal.

Bad food choices, over eating and constant grazing causes frequent spikes in blood sugar leading to constant influxes of insulin. This causes cells to build up a resistance to its effects.

Now less effective at promoting cells to absorb glucose, blood sugar levels stay high. This means more insulin is needed. It also causes the body to assume the cells are full and start storing what it thinks is excess glucose as glycogen and fat. It is not only the high rates of insulin that now prevent weight loss but its constant presence. Under these circumstances it's common to have high fasted insulin levels. This means even when you're not eating you're in storage mode. Under these circumstances you will almost always be in a state of storage….Even if you diet and exercise.

Symptoms of possible Insulin Resistance
- Fatigue
- Extra weight in the middle
- Elevated fasting blood sugar
- Acne
- Fatty liver disease
- Sugar and carb cravings
- Feeling hangry
- High blood pressure
- Fluid retention, swelling in ankles
- High blood pressure
- Trouble concentrating

The bottom line is…
During the fasted period blood sugar levels drop. This triggers Human Growth Hormone (HGH) and glucagon secretion which actively work to break down stored glucagon and fat. This break in insulin secretion also helps to reverse insulin resistance. Under these conditions you will promote hormone health and can gradually bring down your calories when and if you plateau avoiding massive metabolic responses to promote long lasting weight loss.

BEFORE YOU START….

I'm frequently asked if there are any special protocols you should undertake before starting IF. In all honesty? 16:8 is probably the easiest method for beginners and in my view doesn't require any build up phases or special considerations.

However, just like any other health and fitness program you should seek the guidance of a relevant professional and **consult your doctor before starting any nutrition or exercise program including an intermittent fasting cycle.**

Also…..If you

- **Are pregnant or nursing**
- **Have an eating disorder such as anorexia or bulimia**
- **Are under 18**
- **Have medication dependent diabetes (Consult your doctor on this one)**
- **Have liver or kidney disease**
- **Are malnourished, anaemic, exhausted or frail**

Do Not Fast

Again, always consult your doctor before starting any diet, eating pattern or exercise program but especially if you are on medication or suffer with sickness or disease including extremely high blood pressure.

Chapter 2: Selecting An Ideal Eating Window

For the 16:8 method you'll need to choose an eight hour eating window.

The number one rule is **- YOUR WINDOW MUST SUIT YOUR CURRENT LIFE STYLE.**

I have often witnessed clients attempting to follow an eating window that simply does not suit their lifestyle.

An example is a client trying to follow a window that finished in the afternoon because a study she read suggested closing your window at 3pm speeds up the weight loss process.

The problem? My client had a habit of late night snacking once her children were in bed. She also found it weird not eating dinner with her family at night. These two factors caused her to break her fast more often than optimal.

In her case, 7am – 3pm did not suit her life style causing her to fail. Whatever extra benefit she believed this window would give her was obsolete because her adherence to 16:8 was minimal. It was far better for her to start her window later in the day to accommodate dinner with her family and at least keep the late night snacking within her eating window.

Now….she could stick to her window, start getting results and work on breaking the habit of late night snacking.

Using the following questions select your ideal window.

When are you most likely to exercise discipline?
If you find it hard saying no to food after dinner then you should most probably accommodate this period during your eating window. There will be time to work on bad habits later. For now it's important you can stick to your window. Most people find it easier skipping breakfast and starting the eating window later in the day. This doesn't mean you have to do the same but it's worth noting.

Try to incorporate your eating window around the times you feel you are more likely to cave to cravings, outside influences and stress.

What time of the day are you most busy?
Ever been hungry but too busy to eat? Did you find it weird that when you finally got the chance you weren't really hungry anymore? It's far easier to stay the course if you stay busy. For that reason, the busiest part of your day should fall within your fasted window whenever possible.

When are you able to prepare meals?
There's no point trying to start an eating window when you have no food.
Workout when you will actually be able to prepare food. You could also consider food prepping the night before. Don't get caught out having to buy fast food once you're eating window starts due to lack of time management!

Do you struggle with cravings at certain times of the day?
Do you need a sugar hit at 3pm? Or perhaps like my client you struggle with late night snacking. At the start it's best to incorporate these times within your eating window. Discipline can be built over time but often these cravings are the result of lack of nutrition. While you get on top of old habits best not tempt fate. Rome wasn't built in a day!

FAQ

Does it really matter what time of day your eating window is?
Studies have shown eating late at night is not ideal for weight loss. In fact some showed those who work night shift are more likely to suffer from diseases such as diabetes due to unfavourable sleeping and eating patterns. In my experience however, it seems far more important that you have a window you can stick to first and foremost. Adherence is key!

How strict should you be with your window?
For favourable hormone adaptations the timing of food and sleep is important. Your circadian clock (body clock) has a major influence on hormone secretion and is set according to eating and sleeping patterns. For this reason it's optimal to be quite regimented with your eating window. However life is busy! There will be times where this just isn't feasible. Below are some guidelines you can use.

- Begin your eating window within 30 minutes each side of your intended start time. For example, If you intend to eventually have a window that starts at 10am. Beginning to eat anywhere between 9.30am – 10.30am is fine.

- The same rule applies at the end of your window. If you intend to have a window that ends at 6pm having your last meal anywhere between 5.30pm and 6.30pm is fine.

Sometimes life won't permit you to fast a full 16 hours but its ok!! Don't stress out or think it won't work. Studies have shown newbies can start to get favourable hormone adaptation from a nine hour fast!

I want this but I also want to live!! What should I do in the weekends and on social occasions?

ADHERENCE IS KEY! Therefore as a beginner you're going to have to cut yourself some slack. Remember, the goal here is sustainable long term weight loss and health. With that in mind here's my advice.

Tip 1 – Don't Fast On Saturdays/ Days you have an occasion. Practicing 16:8 5-6 days per week is more than enough for positive hormonal adaptations and results.

Tip 2 – Start your fasting window later in the weekends/ nights you have social events. Moving your window around one to two days a week won't matter or effect your body clock in a major way.

Step 1

Using the information outlined in this chapter select your ideal eating window.

Make sure you have a window you can stick to for at least five days before moving on to the remaining steps.

Building good habits is key to success. There's no point moving forward without first adapting to an ideal eating window.

Macronutrients

Macronutrients refer to the big molecules needed to sus[tain] important functions of life. You would most probably know of the[m] as protein, carbohydrates and fats. To help you reach your goals I've condensed information surrounding macronutrients into easy to follow steps and guidelines.

Selecting and maintaining an eating window will certainly put you on the path to health, weight loss and favourable hormone patterns; but <u>what</u> you eat is just as important as <u>when</u> you eat. Although IF should be treated as an eating pattern not a diet, for optimal health, results and energy levels food choices are crucial. Simply eating whatever you want, as much as you want with in an 8 hour window may not yield the results you're after. You can however, still enjoy the foods you love within your window and get great results but you can't just live on cake with no vegetables!

The great thing? You can improve health with a variety of small changes to the food you already eat! This means when you do eat your favourite guilty pleasures the effects on results will be minimal. Keep reading to find out how.

Protein

Known as the building blocks of life, protein is broken down into amino acids and then absorbed into the blood stream to be used by cells.

How much should you eat?
Consuming too much protein can hinder weight loss as excess protein stimulates gluconeogenesis. Basically the extra amino acids are turned into glucose (sugar) and have the potential to be stored. Not enough protein however could impact muscle preservation (1). Following are some equations you can use to calculate how much you should be consuming.

If you haven't got on the exercise band wagon yet
0.8g of protein per kilo of TARGET body weight should fulfill your daily requirements (2).

Example: Joan weighs 85kg but has a goal weight of 75kg.
0.8 x 75 = 60

Joan's ideal daily intake of protein is 60g. Joan would now make sure she had at least 60g of protein per day to avoid deficiency, but eat no more to avoid weight gain.

You are between the ages of 40 – 50
As we get older we naturally lose muscle mass. To help prevent this and maintain quality of life 1g per kilo of body weight is recommended (2).

Example: Joan turns 40 and weighs 75kg.
1 x 75 = 75g

Joan would now consume 75g of protein per day even though when she was younger she used to consume less.

You exercise regularly
Those who train are naturally going to require more protein; especially when incorporating resistance training (weights). The recommended intake is 1.2g – 1.5g of protein a day (2).

Example: Joan regularly does resistance training and has a goal weight of 70kg.

1.2 x 70 = 84
1.5 x 70 = 105

Joan's ideal daily intake would be between 84g – 105g to support lean muscle growth and repair.

Quick Guide To Eating Protein

After determining your daily needs, use the guidelines below for maximal results.

1. Eat as snacks – Protein suppresses hunger by lowering levels of ghrelin – the hunger hormone. Choosing to consume snacks higher in protein and lower in sugar has been shown to decrease appetite and cause people to eat less later in the day (3).

2. Space consumption out over the course of the day. Protein has been shown to raise metabolism because of the energy required for processing. Consuming it over the course of the day could help you burn more calories (3).

3. Consume slow digesting protein before bed – Taking a slow digesting protein such as casein powder before bed has been linked to a higher metabolism during the night. It also helps with muscle growth and recovery by supplying a steady stream of amino acids for the body to use while you sleep. If protein consumption upsets your stomach you may want to skip this tip.

4. Before or after resistance training – Consuming small amounts of protein immediately before or after resistance training has been shown to result in greater strength and muscle growth (4).

5. After cardio training – It has been found when doing cardio, It is better to consume your protein after the workout (4).

FAQ

How much protein should be consumed in each meal?
Divide your ideal intake (worked out with the equation mentioned earlier) by the amount of meals you eat. This will suffice for the beginner. Beware this may change if you attempt keto, OMAD (one meal a day) or any other fasting or low carb regimes.

Do BCCA's break a fast?
Yes. BCCA's stands for branch chain amino acids. This is the micronutrient digested from protein and is insulinogenic.

Should I take protein powder?
This is optional, but there a few reasons you might consider taking protein supplements:

1. You struggle to get your recommended intake through food
2. It's a handy way to promote muscle growth straight after a workout
3. Slow digesting powders like casein are popular before bed to help stimulate repair and growth through the night.
4. It stops some people cheating as it feels like a cheat

If I'm going to take protein powder which are best?
In most cases any natural grass feed whey powders are fine. Been fast digesting, they are great with a piece of fruit after a workout. Casein is a slow digesting equivalent best taken before bed.

Is Isolate protein powder better than regular?
Isolate is a cleaner purer protein source. In most cases it's unnecessary to spend the extra money this will cost you. Spend it on avocados!!

I'm Vegan. Is there any protein powders I can have?
Yes! Pea isolate is a favourite among vegans but shop around there are definitely vegan options out there.

Step 2

From the equations outlined in this chapter, select the equation that best describes your current activity level. Use this and the guidelines section to consume protein in an optimal way for weight loss.

To track protein I suggest using the mobile app my fitness pal. Simply track your intake for a week to get a gauge of what your ideal amount looks like. After that estimating will suffice.

Always Consult Your Doctor When Changing Your Diet

Chapter 4: Carbohydrates

The severe restriction exercised when most people try to diet could be the cause of plateaus, sugar cravings and eventual relapse. It's important to realise not all carbohydrates are equal. If you're serious about weight loss it's time to learn what, when and how you should incorporate these bad boys into your diet. Carbohydrates are typically classified as two types…

Monosaccharides (Simple Carbs)
They are the simplest form of carbohydrate and cannot be broken down any further (Example glucose). Every carbohydrate you consume is digested into simple sugars before they're absorbed by the body, regardless of what you ate. It could be chocolate or brown pasta but it'll end up simple carbs in the end. Some foods don't need to be broken down very much and enter the body predominantly simple. They are absorbed quickly and impact blood sugar and insulin levels drastically.

Polysaccharides (Complex carbs)
Unlike simple carbs they have more than two sugar groups linked together. Complex carbs take time to be broken down into mono saccharides for absorption meaning they make their way into the blood stream much slower. This has less impact on blood sugar levels and insulin secretion.
Examples

Simple Carbohydrate	**Complex Carbohydrate**
Fruit	Potato
Table sugar	Rice
Processed foods	Oatmeal
Milk	Quinoa
Corn syrups	Beans

Even foods categorized under the same carb type are not created equal. A piece of fruit is obviously better than eating chocolate. The difference is fruit carries nutrients that chocolate does not. This is what the term "empty calories" relates to.

Resistant Starch

Resistant starch acts like a soluble fiber in that it is resistant to digestion. Rather than been absorbed as glucose (sugar) like other types of carbs it is broken down into short chain fatty acids by intestinal bacteria. These can be absorbed into the body via the colon or used by good digestive bacteria for energy. Since resistant starches aren't fully digested, we absorb less calories from them than other carbohydrate options. In fact we may only absorb up to 2 calories per gram from resistant starches as opposed to 4 calories per gram from other carbohydrates (5).

3 Reasons To Eat Resistant Starch

1. When taking resistant starches the effect on blood glucose levels are extremely minimal. This promotes insulin sensitivity. You would still eat these during the fasted window as most foods will not be 100% resistant starch.

2. Resistant starches promote digestive health by turning into small chain fatty acids which are consumed by good bacteria. This helps stop sugar cravings.

3. They help you stay lean because you absorb less calories

Resistant Starch Examples

Green Bananas
Green and yellow bananas are considered a healthy form of carbohydrate because they provide nutrients such as vitamin B6 (energy booster). The difference is as bananas ripen the resistant starch transforms into simple sugars like fructose (remember those mono saccharides??).
Therefore, to feed your gut bacteria and help you lose weight by avoiding a spike in insulin aim to buy green bananas (6).

Oats
Oatmeal flakes contain antioxidants and pack a whopping 3.2g of resistant starch per 100g. Oats are best eaten when cooked and left to cool overnight. This increases the resistant starch content even more! (6)

Potatoes
These bad boys are usually the first to get the chop when anyone diets; but as a beginner this can be hard. You've given up all your favourite junk, sweet drinks, pastas and bread. Oh the torment! You may find yourself looking at your plate longing for a potato or two. Will you're in luck. There is a way you can enjoy the odd spud and make sure he's not hindering your results. Cooling potatoes for at least a couple of hours after cooking them significantly increases the amount of resistant starch in them. They are also a good source of potassium. If you hit a plateau you can slowly cut them out. Choose to bake, boil or roast rather than fry potatoes as frying can cause the starch to become harmful (6) (7).

Rice
Just like potatoes, rice has significantly more resistant starch when cooled. It can also be convenient to cook in massive quantities for the week ahead. You can slowly cut this back should results stop (6).

Sweet potato or Yams
Just like potatoes it is better to bake, boil or roast sweet potato. A nutrient dense food with the potential to stop sugar cravings makes this resistant starch an awesome addition to the dinner plate. Cooked and cooled for at least a few hours will once again increase resistant starch. Are you noticing a pattern yet? (7)

Quick Guide To Eating Carbohydrates

If you've had trouble losing weight in the past it could be due to consuming to many simple carbohydrates in low-nutrient high energy foods such as chocolate, soda, biscuits ect….

But have you ever cut those foods out only to see little to no results? This could be because carbohydrates you thought "healthy" are still messing with your hormones. Does this mean you should avoid simple carbohydrates? No. You just have to be wiser about when you eat them so you can use the insulin spike they give you to your advantage.

1. <u>Eat With Protein</u> - If you do eat simple carbohydrates, consume them with a source of protein. This slows absorption having less effect on blood sugar levels. For example a piece of fruit and a small handful of almonds.

2. <u>To Break a Fast</u> - If your goal is to build lean muscle, break your fast with a simple carbohydrate and a fast digesting protein to stop any break down of muscle that may be happening from the fast. An example of this would be an apple and a protein shake or BCCA'S. The sugar from the apple mixed with the protein will spike insulin refilling glycogen stores and pushing the protein into your muscles for growth and repair.

3. <u>Pre – workout</u> - Consuming simple carbs 20-30 minutes before a workout will give your cells an abundance of readily available energy to get you through the grind. It is less likely to be converted to fat at this stage.

4. <u>Post - Workout</u> - Consuming simple carbs after a workout with fast digesting protein promotes insulin to push amino acids into the muscles for repair while restocking glycogen stores.

5. <u>Do Not Eat Simple Carbohydrates Before Bed</u> – High energy intake right before bed can effect sleep which in turn effects results. Poor quality sleep effects your weight loss hormones just as much as eating crap does!

6. <u>Aim to eat complex carbs wherever possible</u> out-side of the times mentioned above. Their slow digesting nature means they won't impact blood sugar and insulin as much as simple carbs promoting sustainable energy to help avoid sugar cravings and energy crashes.

7. <u>Increase The Resistant Starch Content Wherever Possible</u> – Using methods such as cooking and cooling oats overnight means you're going to absorb less calories and feed those healthy stomach bacteria in your digestive tract stopping sugar cravings. It's well worth the effort!

Eating carbohydrates using these guidelines minimizes the chances of insulin promoting it to be stored as fat. Guidelines 2 – 4 use insulin spikes to allow protein to be absorbed quickly to promote muscle growth and repair. These guidelines were not formed for the ketogenic approach to fasting.

Step 3

Your third step will be to replace one of the carbohydrates you currently eat for one of the resistant starch types. You'll also use the guidelines at the end of the chapter to determine when you should eat certain carbohydrates.

Always Consult Your Doctor When Changing Your Diet

Chapter 5: Healthy Fats

With fats still been widely blamed for obesity and heart disease a lot of people find it hard to comprehend that eating fat doesn't automatically equal fat around the midline, nor does it sentence you to heart disease and diabetes. So where does this line of thought come from?

When researchers first discovered saturated fat raises cholesterol they (with good intention) recommended lower fat intake was beneficial. Unfortunately there was a huge flaw… they only measured <u>total</u> cholesterol. As you'll learn next there is actually more than one marker for cholesterol and they're not equal in their effects on heart health (8).

<u>LDL Cholesterol & HDL Cholesterol</u>
Before continuing it's important to note LDL "Bad" and HDL "Good" cholesterols are not actually cholesterol but refer to the proteins used to transport cholesterol in the blood stream. The differences are below (9).

- LDL "Bad" is smaller and lower in density meaning it can easily penetrate arterial walls. These particles are also more likely to be oxidized. Both are scenarios that drive heart disease.

- HDL "Good" particles are bigger and fluffy meaning they don't penetrate arterial walls as easily.

Even though saturated fat elevates over all cholesterol and is linked to higher LDL levels short term, it has been found there are many different sub types of LDL that don't in fact increase risk of heart disease. So where is the problem? The lynching of saturated fat ended up demonizing all fats. People started eliminating fat wherever possible and getting their calories from refined carbohydrates. The obesity crisis is probably indirectly linked to the low fat movement and the rise of processed foods in the average diet. Just like carbohydrates, not all fats are created equal. Studies have now shown that replacing saturated and trans-fat with unsaturated fat <u>NOT</u> refined carbohydrates is what leads to better heart health and weight loss (10).

Following is some basic information you can use to get the most out of fat while fasting.

Saturated Fat
As mentioned earlier the criticism saturated fat has faced seems to be unjustified with many studies showing it can in fact lower the risk of heart disease long term. Found in meat and dairy products, you'll also find saturated fat in products like coconut oil. Saturated fats are solid at room temperature and is the safest choice for cooking as they have a higher melting point and less chance of turning into trans-fat. Outside of cooking the general consensus is that swapping saturated fat for unsaturated fat where ever possible, NOT refined carbohydrates leads to heart health and weight loss (10, 11, 12).

Unsaturated Fat
Unsaturated fats consist of mono and polyunsaturated fats. With the goal of keeping things simple, I'm going to skip the rant about double bonds ect. All you need to know is their molecular structure is what makes them different. Basically they go together a little different and have a slightly different shape (11,12).

> Monounsaturated Fat: Deemed one of the healthy fats, monounsaturated fat can be found in plant foods such as avocado, nuts and vegetable oil (11,12, 13). Be advised cooking with monounsaturated fat is not ideal as they become hydrogenised under heat. (Trans fat).

Examples: Avocado, Olive oil, Nuts and seeds

> Polyunsaturated: Polyunsaturated fats include essential fatty acids such as omega- 3 and omega -6. These fats are important for brain function and cell growth and must be consumed as they are not made by the body (14).

Examples: Walnuts, Fish, Sunflower seeds, fish oil tablets

Trans Fat

Trans fat is a type of unsaturated fat that occurs in small amounts in nature. It became widely produced industrially from vegetable fats in the mid-90s. Trans-fat can be found in meat products and is even sold in supplement form (conjugated linoleic acid or CLA). It is deemed safe and even beneficial according to some studies. Where trans-fat becomes problematic is when it is man-made through a process called hydrogenation. This type of trans fat is made by adding hydrogen molecules to vegetable fats which changes its molecular make up. The resulting fat is not only bad for weight loss but bad for health. Best to avoid these where possible (16).

3 Tips To Lower Your Trans Fat Consumption

- Avoid foods that say "hydrogenated" or " partially hydrogenated" on their food label

- Limit processed foods

- Avoid heating unsaturated fats

Quick Guide To Eating Lipids/ Fats

1. Always cook with saturated fat options such as real butter or animal fats as they have a higher melting point (16)

2. Avoid cooking with unsaturated fats such as olive oil as they have a lower melting point (16)

3. Apart from cooking, replace saturated fats and refined carbohydrates with unsaturated fat such as nuts, seeds and fish.

4. Avoid hydrogenated and partially hydrogenated foods

5. Remember the trans-fat found in nature such as the type found in meat and dairy is deemed safe

6. Fish oil tablets contain omega-3s and could be a helpful supplement for health

Step 4

This step involves a few tasks all based around fat consumption.

1. Stop cooking in vegetable, soy bean and corn oils. Use saturated fat such as coconut oil and animal fat for cooking.

2. Check food labels and avoid anything that states the product is "hydrogenated" or "partially hydrogenated".

3. Add a fish oil supplement 3 x a day with food. (Always check with your doctor before supplementing).

These four simple steps (added with the others) can kick start your health in ways you wouldn't believe! Make sure to use the quick guide section of this chapter as well.

Always Consult Your Doctor When Changing Your Diet

Chapter 6: Sugar

Sugar Free Products

Unfortunately "sugar free" or "low sugar" does not always mean a product is safe to consume while fasted - or at all for that matter. It could be harbouring other additives that will indeed spike insulin and undo all that low carb discipline you've been trying to implement. Here are two common additives found in low sugar products. These are also found in foods newbies to keto think are good for them.

- Maltodextrin: A polysaccharide (carbohydrate) that is used to prolong the shelf life of products. It derives from starch so a big no no for all you keto fans. Commonly found in products like bacon so make sure to check the labels!

- Dextrose: A simple sugar derived from corn. Commonly found in processed foods and appears in many low carb protein bars so make sure to check labels. Just because it's a protein bar doesn't make it good for your waist line.

Step 5

ELIMINATE Maltodextrin from your diet……It's just not good for you! If you are trying to go low carb maltodextrin will kill your results and your health! Check food labels and put anything with this stuff in it back on the shelf. If you are going to eat dextrose laden products such as protein bars, be sure to keep them within your eating window.

Sugar Replacements

If you can't kick sugar all together don't worry…. you're not alone! Many transition to a low sugar fasting lifestyle by using replacements at first. Next I've outlined the best replacements and whether they break a fast or not.

Splenda (Sucralose)
Because Splenda contains no calories or carbohydrates it's commonly used as a replacement for sugar when fasting. Be aware, A 2013 study published in the Journal of Toxicology and Environmental Health showed sucralose may indeed effect glucose and insulin levels in both rats and humans. The study showed sucralose reacts with sensors in the GI tract (stomach intestines etc.) that play a role in sweet taste sensation which in turn effects the release of certain hormones. Basically your body has sensors that picks up sweet things and prepares the blood stream to receive them by releasing insulin– yes, tasting something sweet can cause the body to release insulin even if it's not "real sugar". The study also found sucralose is not entirely biologically inert with small amounts been absorbed as it makes its way through the GI tract. I believe Splenda notes 85% is not absorbed (17, 18).

Will it break a fast?
Even though Splenda is 0 calorie it will still effect insulin levels by interacting with sweet sensors and is best avoided outside of your eating window.

Stevia
Been 30 to 150 times sweeter than sugar with far less calories automatically makes it a good choice for sugar substitution. Add the fact it's heat-stable, pH-stable, and doesn't ferment makes replacing sugar with this bad boy a no brainier.

Does Stevia break a fast?
A peer reviewed study found insulin and glucose levels were lowered after a pre load of stevia. I have personally not cited any information suggesting stevia effects the chemo sensors responsible for the sweet sensation leading me to conclude stevia additives in coffee or tea so the beginner can adapt even when fasted is fine (20).

Xylitol

Unlike other sugar substitutes, xylitol occurs naturally and can be extracted from certain vegetables and fruit. It has 40% less calories than sugar but is just as sweet. This makes it a popular replacement among dieters. An article released to educate physicians on recommending sugar replacements had nothing but good things to say about xylitol. It mentions xylitol has little effect on blood sugar levels and insulin secretion and cites its role in a number of benefits from dental health to the prevention of ear infection in young children. The article stated that when consumed this sweetener is gradually metabolized into glucose preventing large blood sugar spikes. It went on to say xylitol is also converted into short chain fatty acids once it reaches the large intestine. So for all you keto fans this is the sweetener you want for your baking! The article also cited it helps curb hunger and the conversion into fatty acids burns most of its original caloric value (20).

Will it break a fast?

Technically it looks like xylitol may indeed break a fast but its effects on blood sugar seem minimal. Switching normal sugar to xylitol in your morning drinks to help you adapt is going to make a tremendous difference. Fast break or not this will lower your intake of normal sugar which of course will help you lose weight! Using this as replacement during the eating window is of course a good idea.

Cinnamon

Known for its anti-diabetic properties, A review of past studies concluded It does indeed lower blood sugar levels and improve insulin sensitivity. Because of this, a little cinnamon in your coffee or tea to get you through may not only keep you sane but boost the reasons your fasting in the first place (21).

Will it break a fast?

Although cinnamon technically breaks a fast with 6 calories per teaspoon, it's health properties outweigh this if you're looking for a way to sweeten your drinks to get you through. If you're really worried about the calories use a quarter teaspoon. Now it's only 1.5 calories.

Step 6

Start replacing table sugar wherever possible for one of the options previously mentioned. Remember, Splenda breaks a fast and is best kept within the eating window. Stevia and xylitol are the preferred choice during the fasted window and cinnamon is a "hybrid" type option when you take into account its health benefits.

Always Consult Your Doctor When Changing Your Diet

Chapter 7: How To Break A Fast

Breaking a fast refers to your first meal. What to eat at this time depends on your personal goal. Following are examples of how to break a fast and when you would implement them.

The Lean Muscle Method
If your goal is to build lean muscle it's important to break your fast with carbohydrates. The sugar will refill glycogen stores and stop any catabolic (break down) effects currently happening from the fast. Consuming your carbohydrate with a fast digesting protein will promote cells to absorb protein in the presence of the insulin spike.

Examples

Simple Carbohydrate	Fast Digesting Protein
Piece of fruit	Whey Protein Shake
Gummy Bears	BCCA's

Pre-Brought
- Post Workout Supplements
- Protein products with dextrose in it

The Supplement Method
If your goal is to burn fat and lose weight, MCT oil is a great way to break a fast. MCT oil will prime the body to burn fat as an energy source throughout the day. Break your fast with the oil and follow with a high fat/protein meal 30 minutes after.

The High Fat/High Protein Method
Another way for optimal fat burning is to simply eat a high fat/protein meal to start your eating window. An example of this would be bacon, eggs and spinach. This would prime the body to keep utilizing fat as a fuel source. Remember to check those labels for maltodextrin!

Examples:

1. Eggs, avocado and spinach
2. Natural full fat yogurt, flaxseeds and sunflower seeds
3. Coconut milk and whey protein
4. Protein pancakes with cream

Step 7

Based on your goal, select your ideal way to break a fast and incorporate it into your lifestyle. If fat loss is your main goal then the supplement or high fat/high protein method is best. If you'd like to build lean muscle then use the lean muscle method.

Always Consult Your Doctor When Changing Your Diet

End Note

Thank you and congratulations! We have come to the end of your 7 step guide. By reading to the end you have proven you are an action taker! This already puts you one step ahead of most people. To truly achieve you must now put the 7 steps outlined in this book to action.
I understand as you progress you will have many more questions.... I certainly did! My aim in this book was to provide basic, easy to follow nutritional information you can implement straight after choosing your eight hour eating window. For any other questions or motivation I suggest you join our FREE Private Facebook support group below;

Link Address: http://bit.ly/fasting_motivation

Here you will find people on the same journey as yourself ready to support, motivate and help each other.

For a bigger overview of hormones, a 30 day guide and other ways outside of fasting to attain hormonal balance for weight loss, I highly suggest you check out the first book in this series –

Intermittent Fasting For Weight Loss: A Beginners Guide to 16:8

You will find a lot more detail on how fasting works and other ways to achieve hormonal imbalance.
This book includes:
- Your first 30 Days
- Why Low-Calorie Diets Make You Fat
- The Best Exercise for Weight Loss
- **The Third most IMPORTANT Factor Other Than Diet & Exercise Most Programs Neglect**

Claim a copy by pasting this link to your browser:
http://bit.ly/fasting_guide

Thank you for reading my book, I look forward to meeting you in the online support group!

Robert Paxton

References

1) Schutz, Y. 2011. Protein turnover, ureagenesis and gluconeogenesis.

Retrieved From: https://www.ncbi.nlm.nih.gov/pubmed/22139560

2) Dorfner, M. 2017. Are you getting too much protein?

Retrieved From: https://newsnetwork.mayoclinic.org/discussion/are-you-getting-too-much-protein/

3) Dominik H. Pesta, Varman T. Samuel. 2014. A high-protein diet for reducing body fat: mechanisms and possible caveats.

Retrieved From: https://www.ncbi.nlm.nih.gov/pmc/articles/PMC4258944/

4) Lemon PW, Berardi JM, Noreen EE. 2002. The role of protein and amino acid supplements in the athlete's diet: does type or timing of ingestion matter?

Retrieved From: https://www.ncbi.nlm.nih.gov/pubmed/12831698

5) Andrew, R. n.d. Resistant starch: What is it? And why is it so good for you?

Retrieved From: https://www.precisionnutrition.com/all-about-resistant-starch

6) Mawer, R. 2016. 9 Foods That Are High in Resistant Starch.

Retrieved From: https://www.healthline.com/nutrition/9-foods-high-in-resistant-starch

7) Scott-Dixon K, Pierre B. n.d. Sweet vs. regular potatoes: Which potatoes are really healthier?

Retrieved From: https://www.precisionnutrition.com/regular-vs-sweet-potatoes

8) Weinberg, S.L. 2004. The diet–heart hypothesis: a critique.

Retrieved From: https://www.sciencedirect.com/science/article/pii/S0735109703016310

9) Gunnars, C. 2017. Saturated Fat: Good or Bad?

Retrieved From: https://www.healthline.com/nutrition/saturated-fat-good-or-bad

10) Packard J, Caslake Muriel, Shepherd J. The role of small, dense low density lipoprotein (LDL): a new look.

Retrieved From: https://www.sciencedirect.com/science/article/pii/S0167527399001072

11) No Author. 2018. The truth about fats: the good, the bad, and the in-between.

Retrieved From: https://www.health.harvard.edu/staying-healthy/the-truth-about-fats-bad-and-good

12) The Nutrition Source. n.d. Types of Fat.

Retrieved From: https://www.hsph.harvard.edu/nutritionsource/what-should-you-eat/fats-and-cholesterol/types-of-fat/

13) Medline Plus. n.d. Facts about monounsaturated fats.

Retrieved From: https://medlineplus.gov/ency/patientinstructions/000785.htm

14) Medline Plus. n.d. Facts about polyunsaturated fats.

Retrieved From: https://medlineplus.gov/ency/patientinstructions/000747.htm

15) Leech, J. 2017. Why Are Trans Fats Bad for You? The Disturbing Truth.

Retrieved From: https://www.healthline.com/nutrition/why-trans-fats-are-bad

16) Retrieved From: http://chemistry.elmhurst.edu/vchembook/551fattyacids.html

17) Migala, J. n.d. What Is Sucralose and Should You Be Eating It?

Retrieved From: http://www.eatingwell.com/article/290901/what-is-sucralose-and-should-you-be-eating-it/

18) Schiffman S, Rother K. Sucralose, A Synthetic Organochlorine Sweetener: Overview of Biological Issues.

Retrieved From: https://www.ncbi.nlm.nih.gov/pmc/articles/PMC3856475/

19) Brady D.M, Copp S. Xylitol Natural Health – Promoting Sweetener.

Retrieved From: https://system.na2.netsuite.com/core/media/media.nl?id=1856&c=ACCT14095&h=d7cc4761455c17541942&_xt=.pdf

20) Stephen D. A, Corby K. M, Hongmei H, Coulon S, Cefalu W, Geiselman P, Williamson D. 2010. Effects of stevia, aspartame, and sucrose on food intake, satiety, and postprandial glucose and insulin levels

Retrieved From: https://www.ncbi.nlm.nih.gov/pmc/articles/PMC2900484/

21) Kirkham S, Akilen R, Sharma S, Tsiami A. 2009. The potential of cinnamon to reduce blood glucose levels in patients with type 2 diabetes and insulin resistance.

Retrieved From: https://www.ncbi.nlm.nih.gov/pubmed/19930003

Made in the USA
Middletown, DE
11 December 2018